Love is the bridge between
You and everything.

Rumi

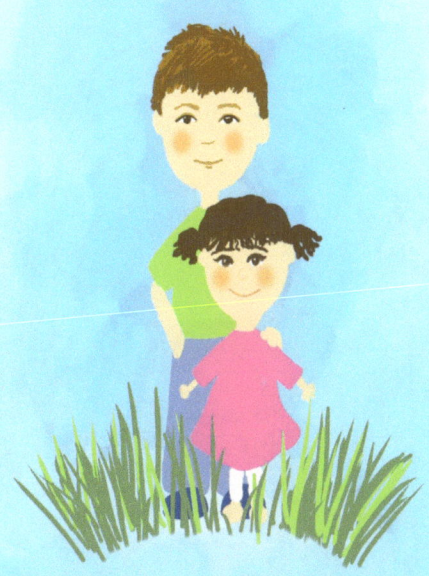

Everyone gets frustrated, sad, or scared sometimes.

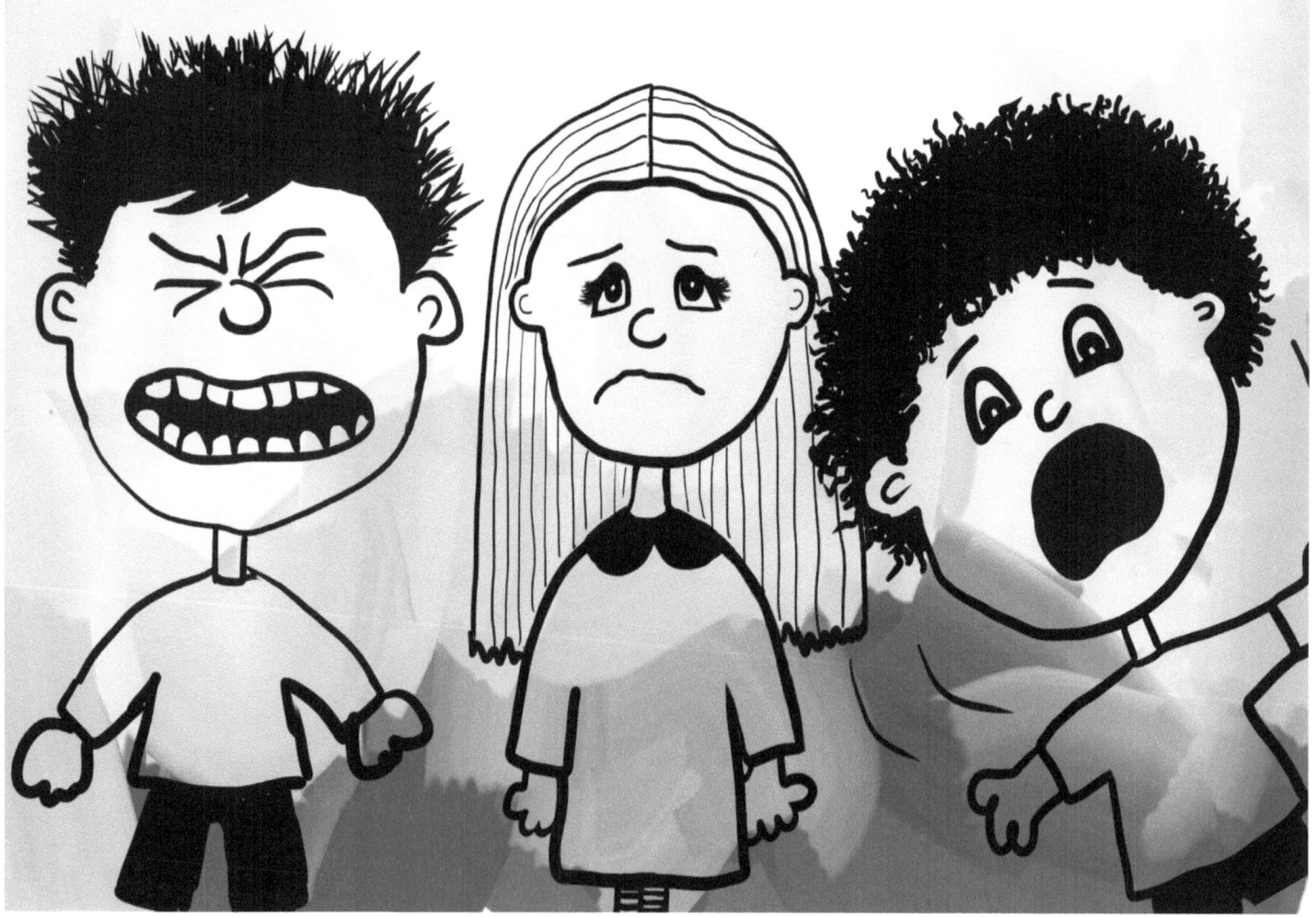

When this happens, remember that there is a place in your heart that is always loving. There you can calm down and find kindness toward yourself and others.

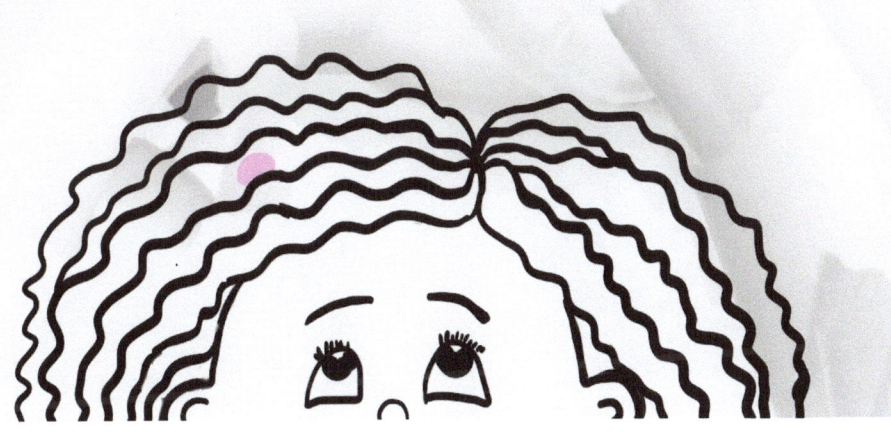

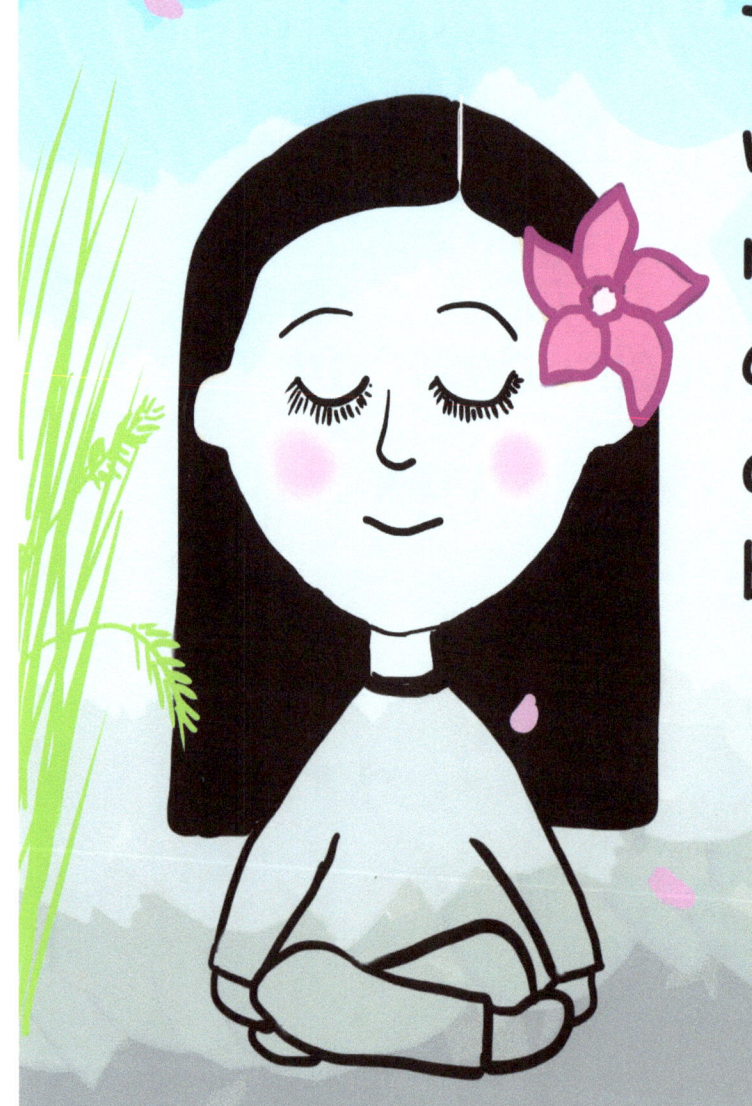

To find this place within your heart, relax, get comfortable, and take a deep breath.

Close your eyes and imagine a tree. This is your loving kindness tree. As you let your love grow your tree will get taller and stronger.

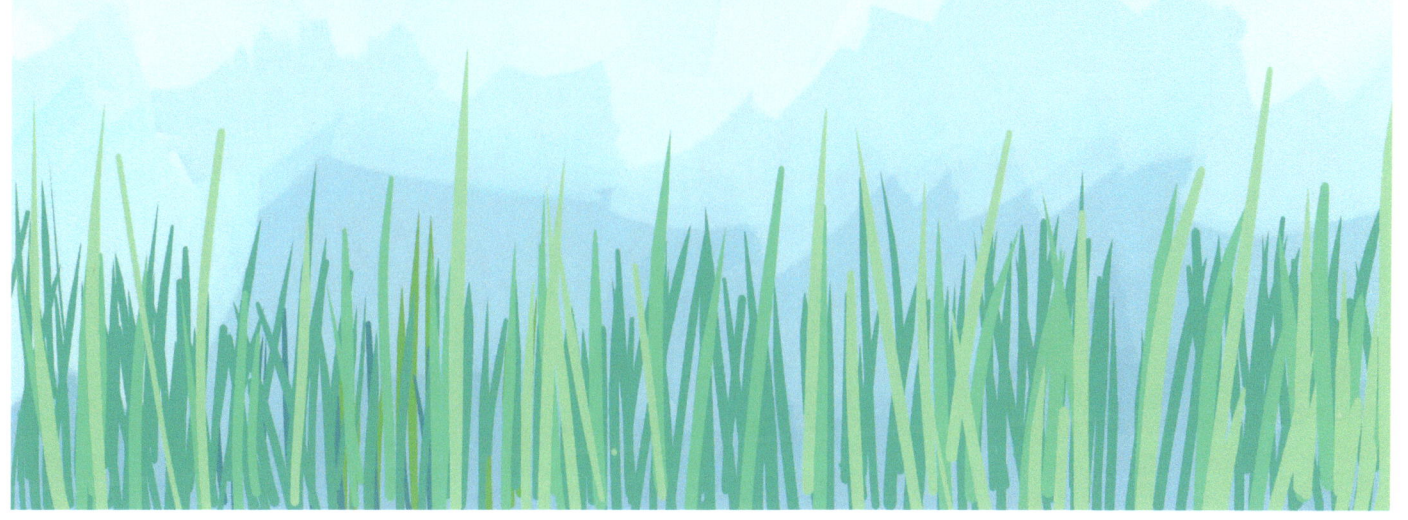

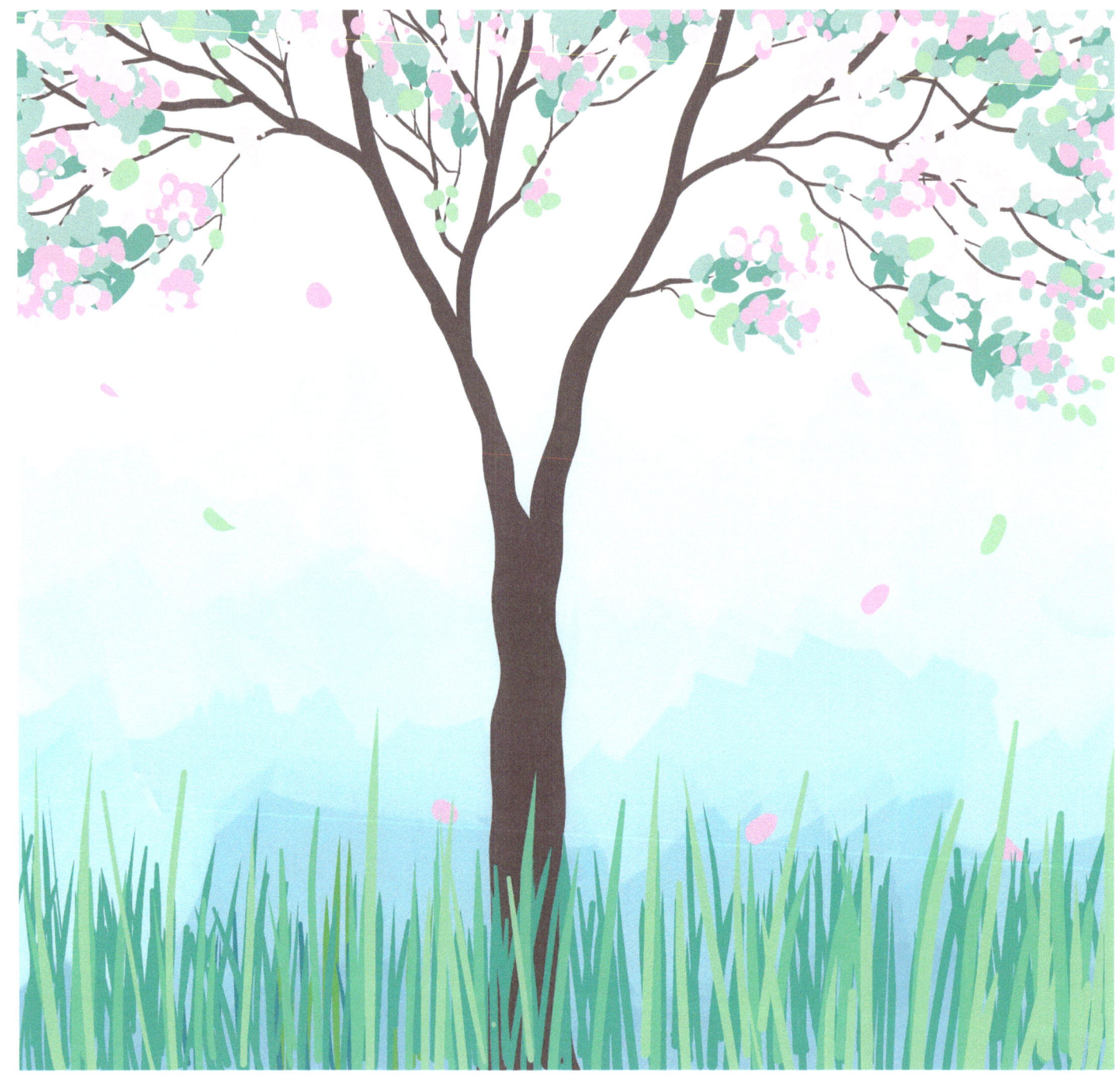

I don't have any friends.

I want to cry but I don't know why.

I wish my dad was here.

Sometimes these clouds are full of sad thoughts.

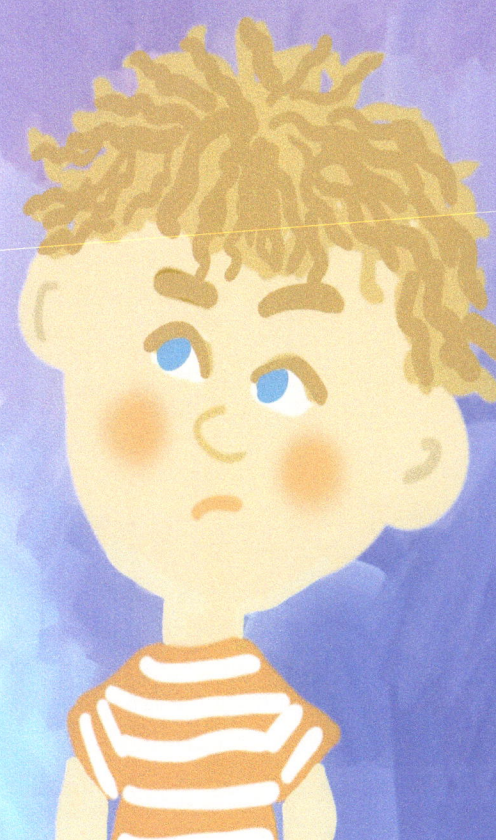

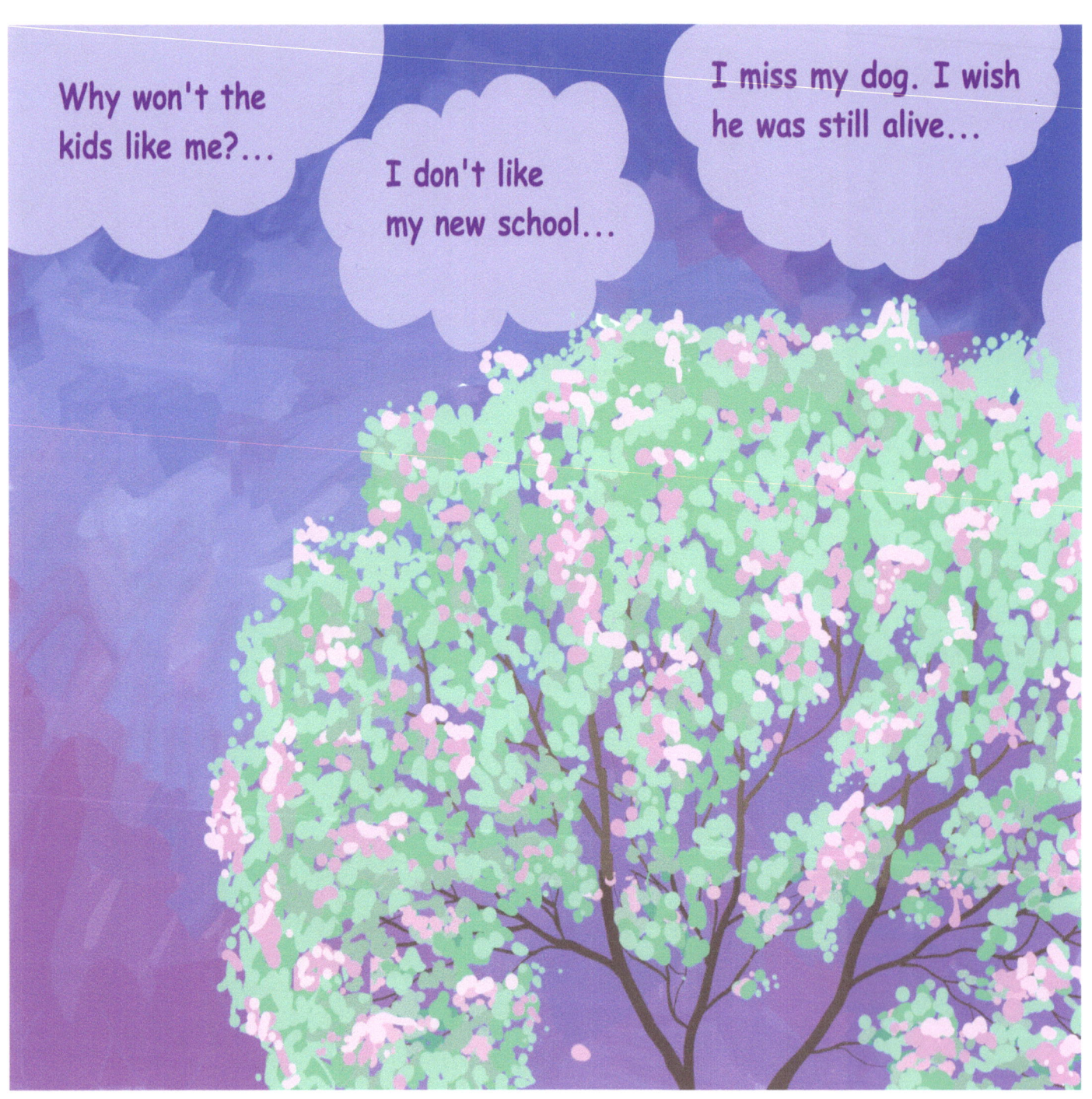

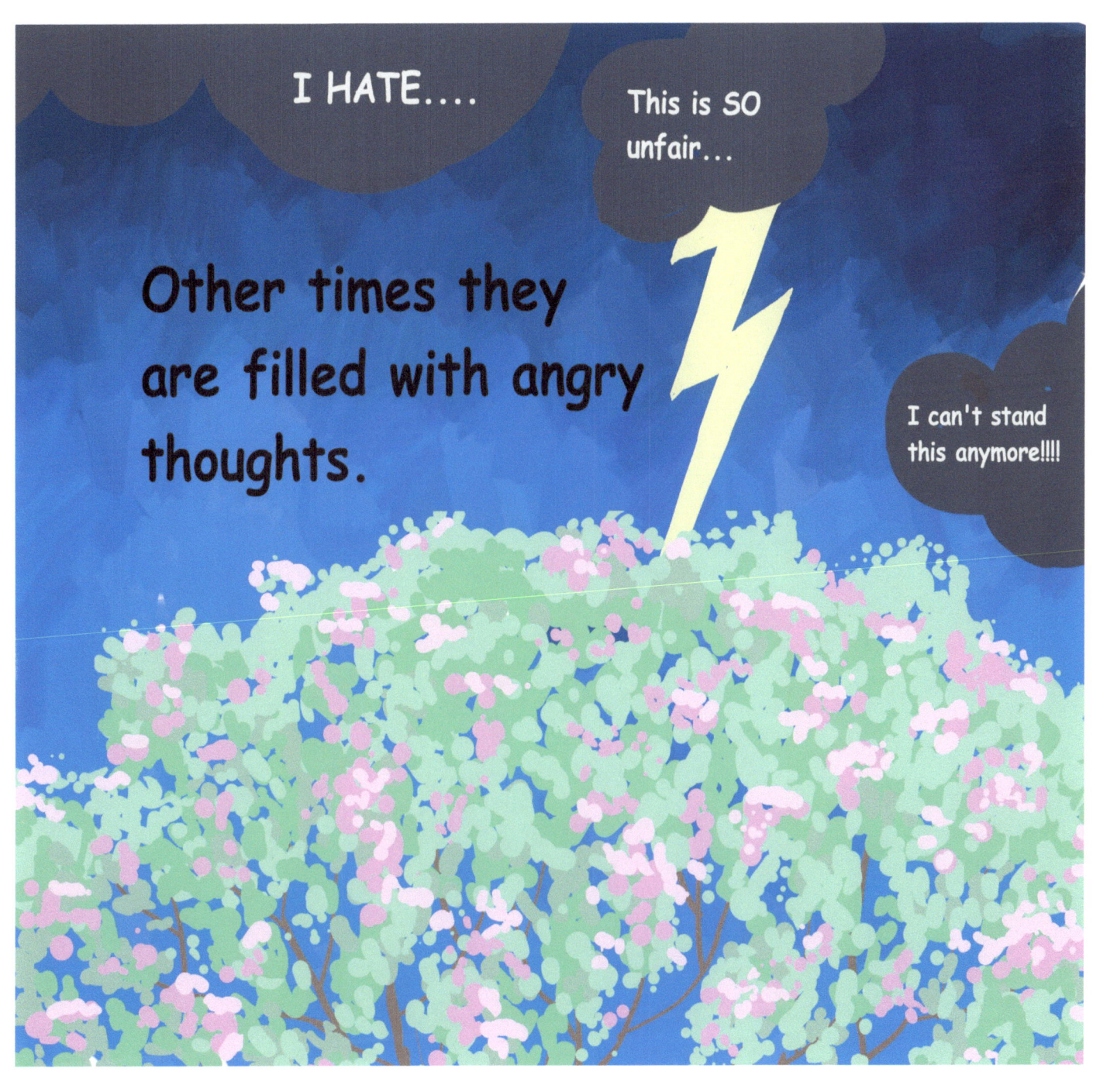

I am so scared of...

I am scared
something
is hiding
in my closet.

Did I do
something
wrong? ...

And sometimes they are full of fears.

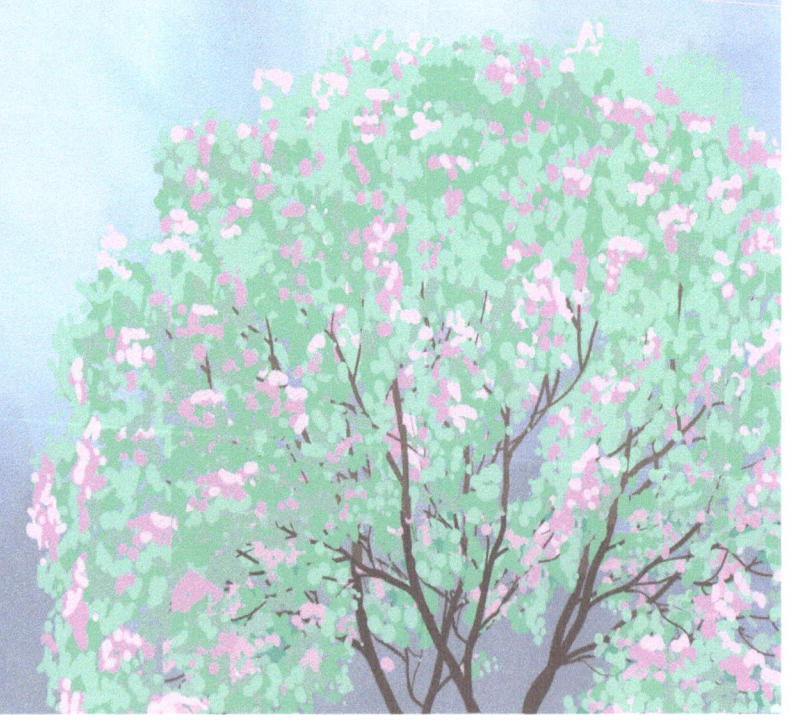

No matter what those feelings or thoughts are your tree stays loving and kind. The clouds come and go.

Now let's see your
tree grow.
Tell yourself...

May I be
healthy and safe.
May I be peaceful.
May I give and
receive love.

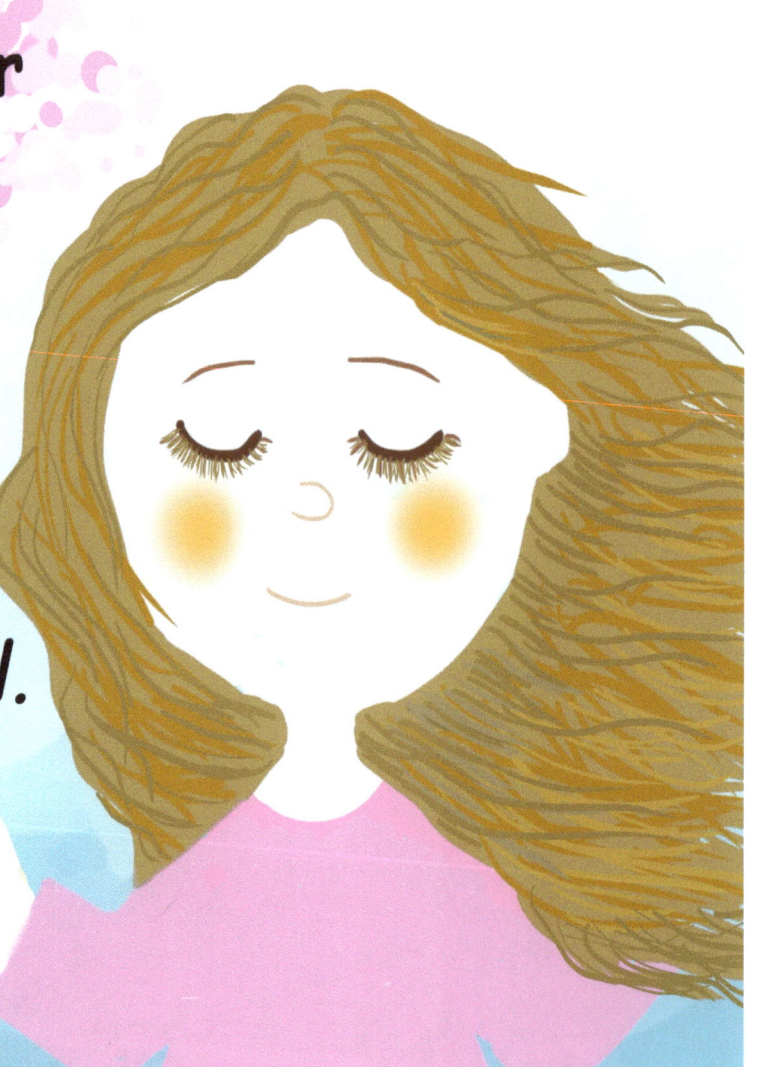

Now wish the same to someone who makes you all warm and happy inside. Tell her or him...

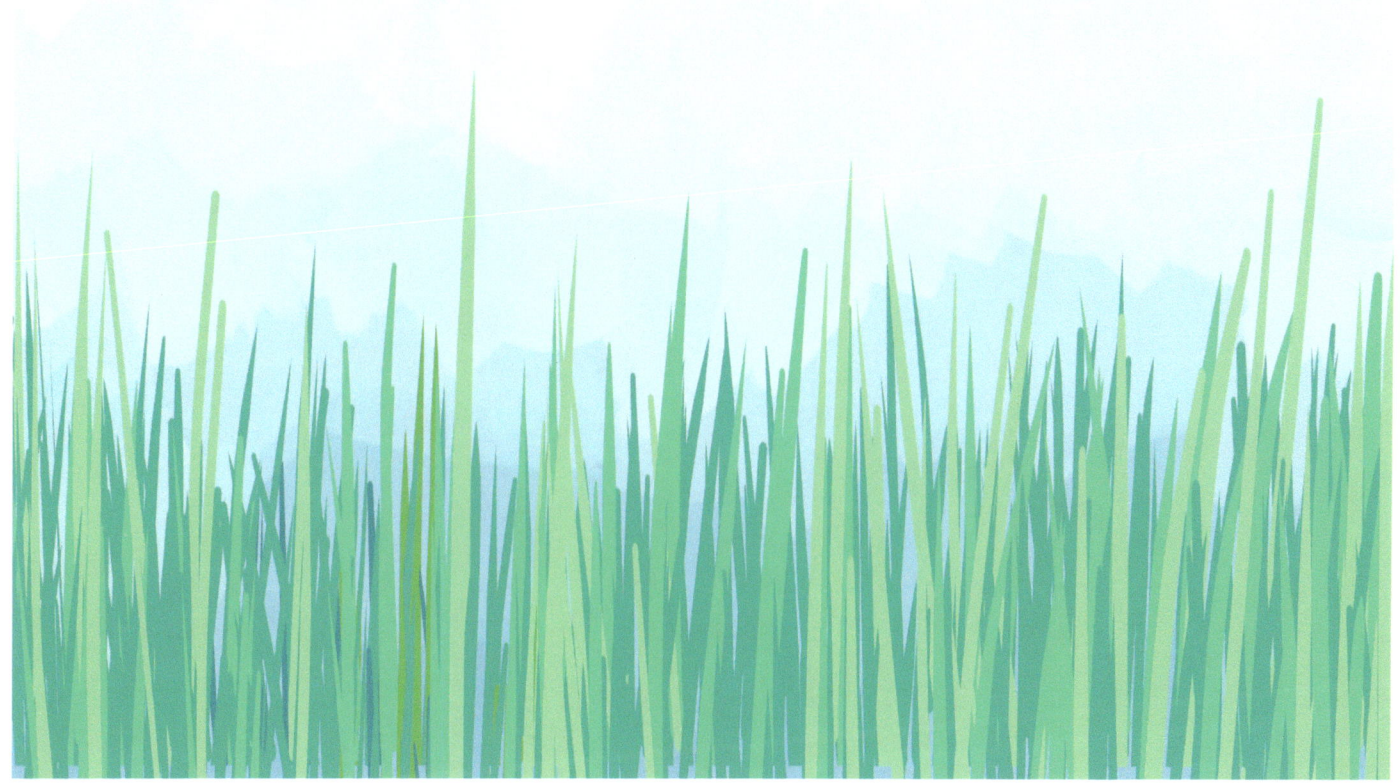

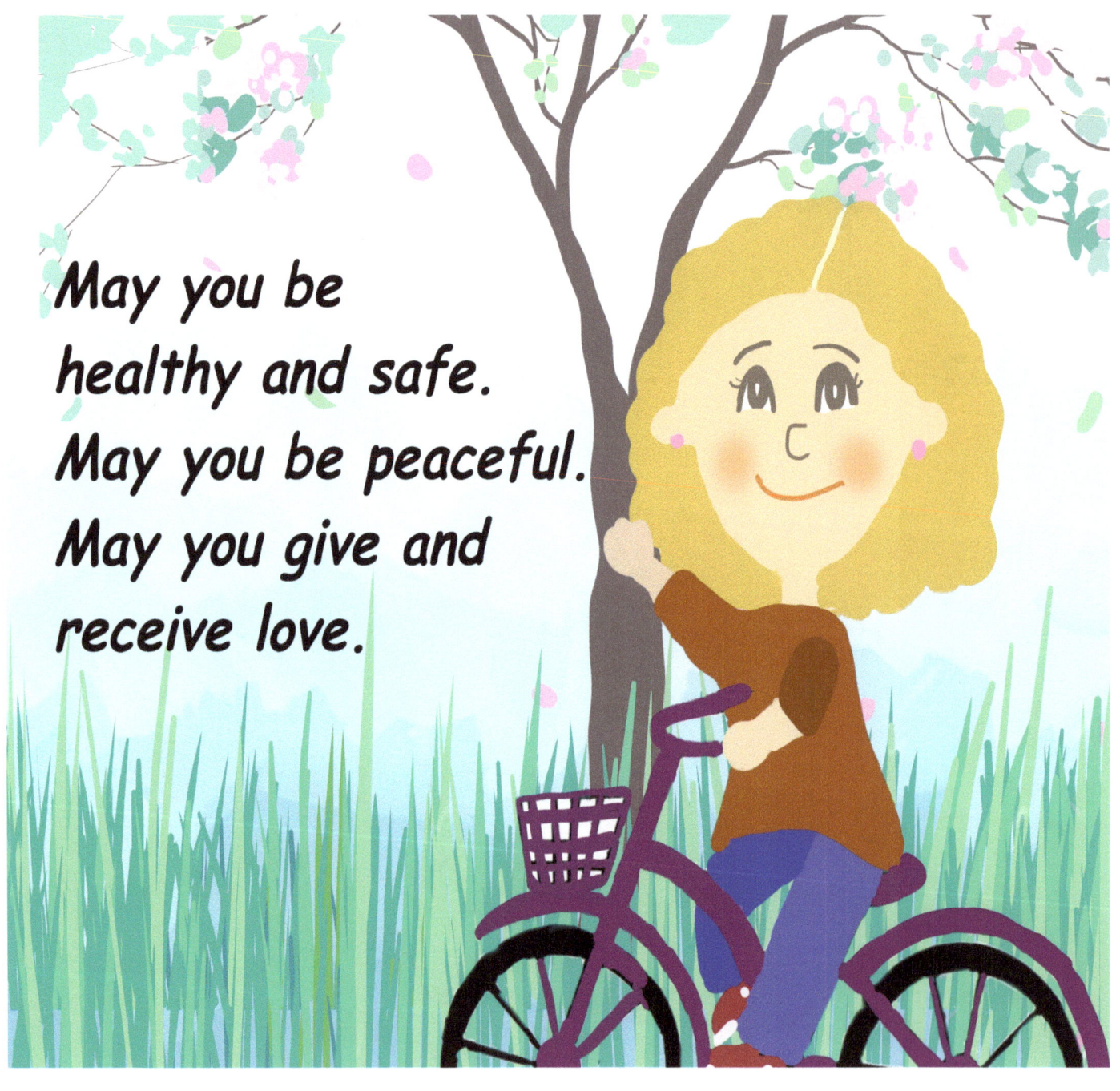

May you be
healthy and safe.
May you be peaceful.
May you give and
receive love.

Imagine someone you know very little.
It could be a neighbor or your friends'
parents.Tell them...

May you be healthy and safe
May you be peaceful.
May you give and receive love.

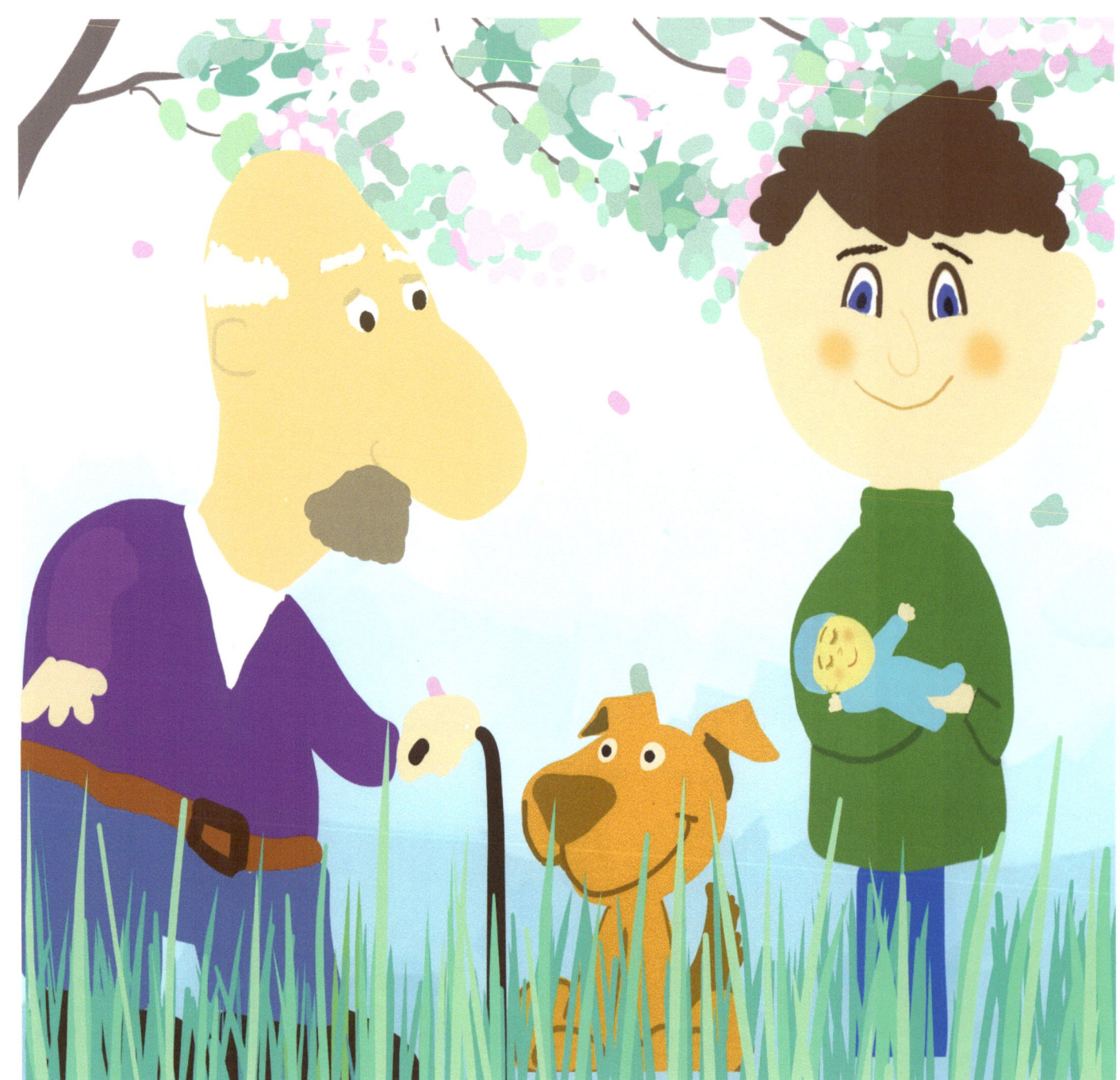

Can you remember someone you had a hard time with a long time ago? Imagine this person and say the words...

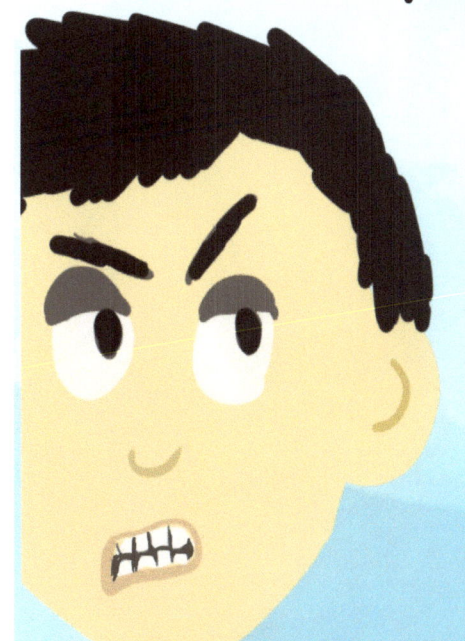

May he or she be healthy and safe. May he or she be peaceful. May he or she give and receive love.

The more people receive
your loving wishes
the taller and stronger
your tree becomes.

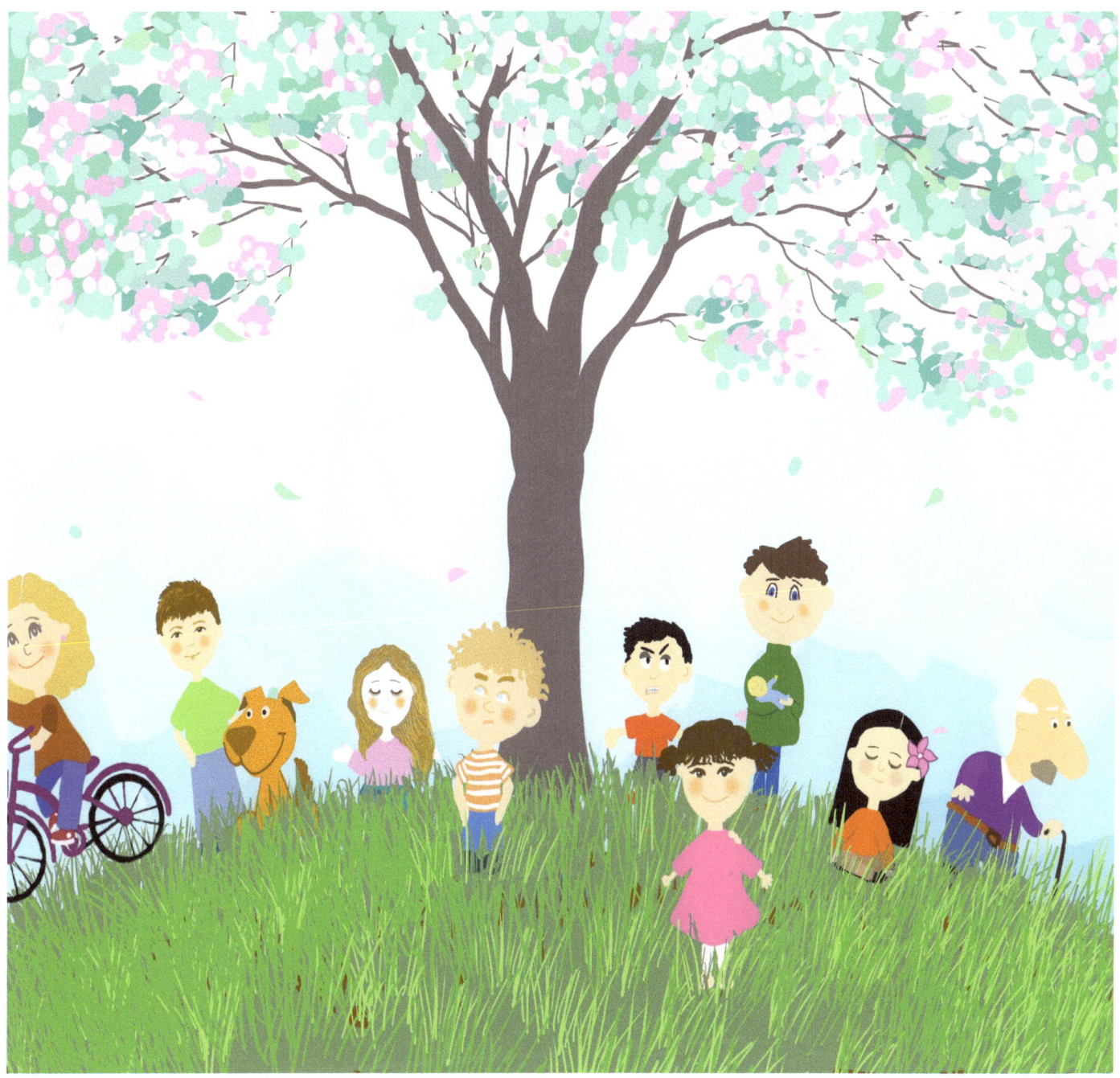

Now share your love with
all the living creatures.

May we all be healthy and safe.
May we all be peaceful.
May we all give and receive love.

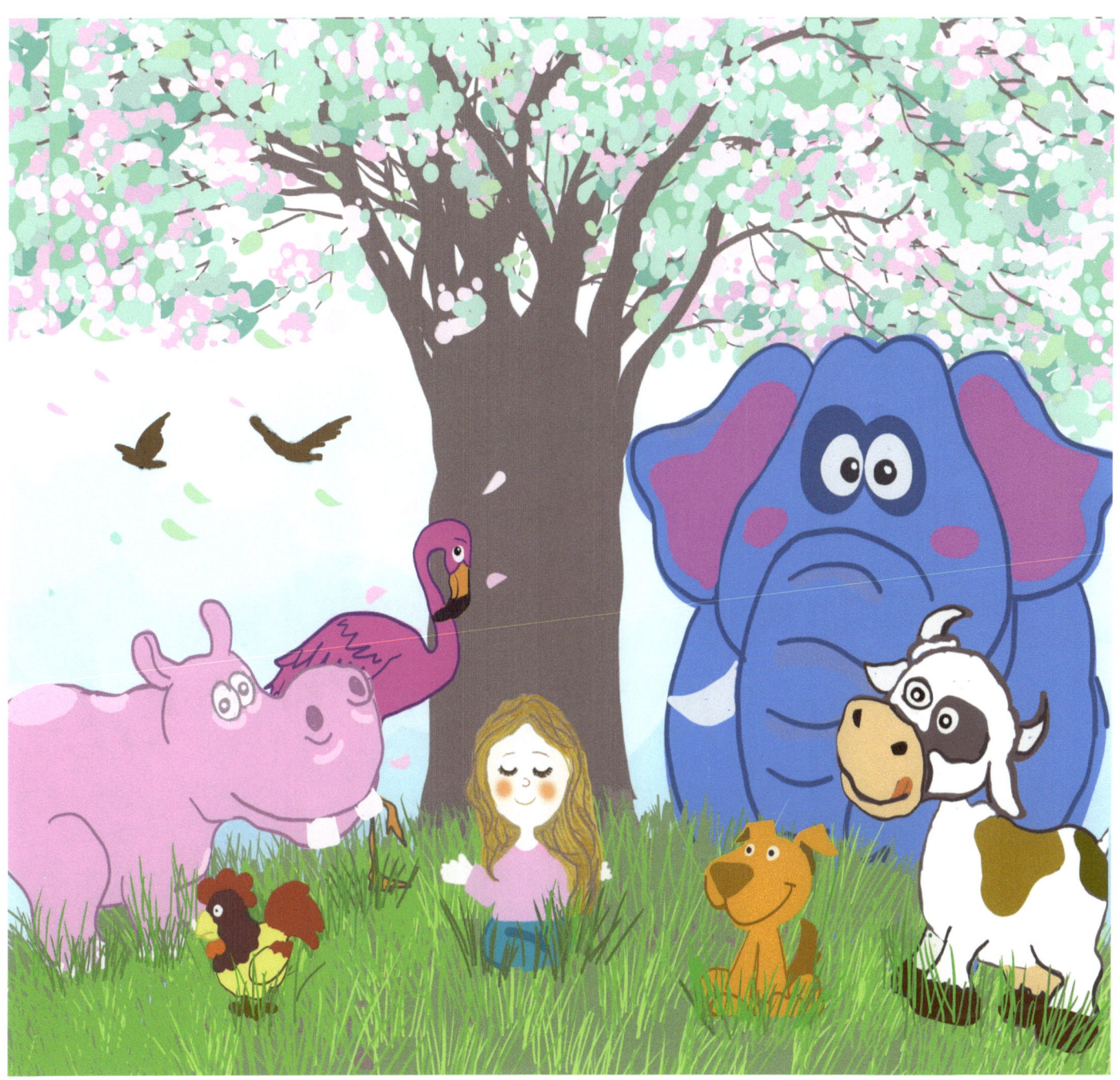

There will be all kinds of
feelings and thoughts in your
life that will come and go.
Be mindful of the journey,
and remember that your place
of inner love is always there
for you.

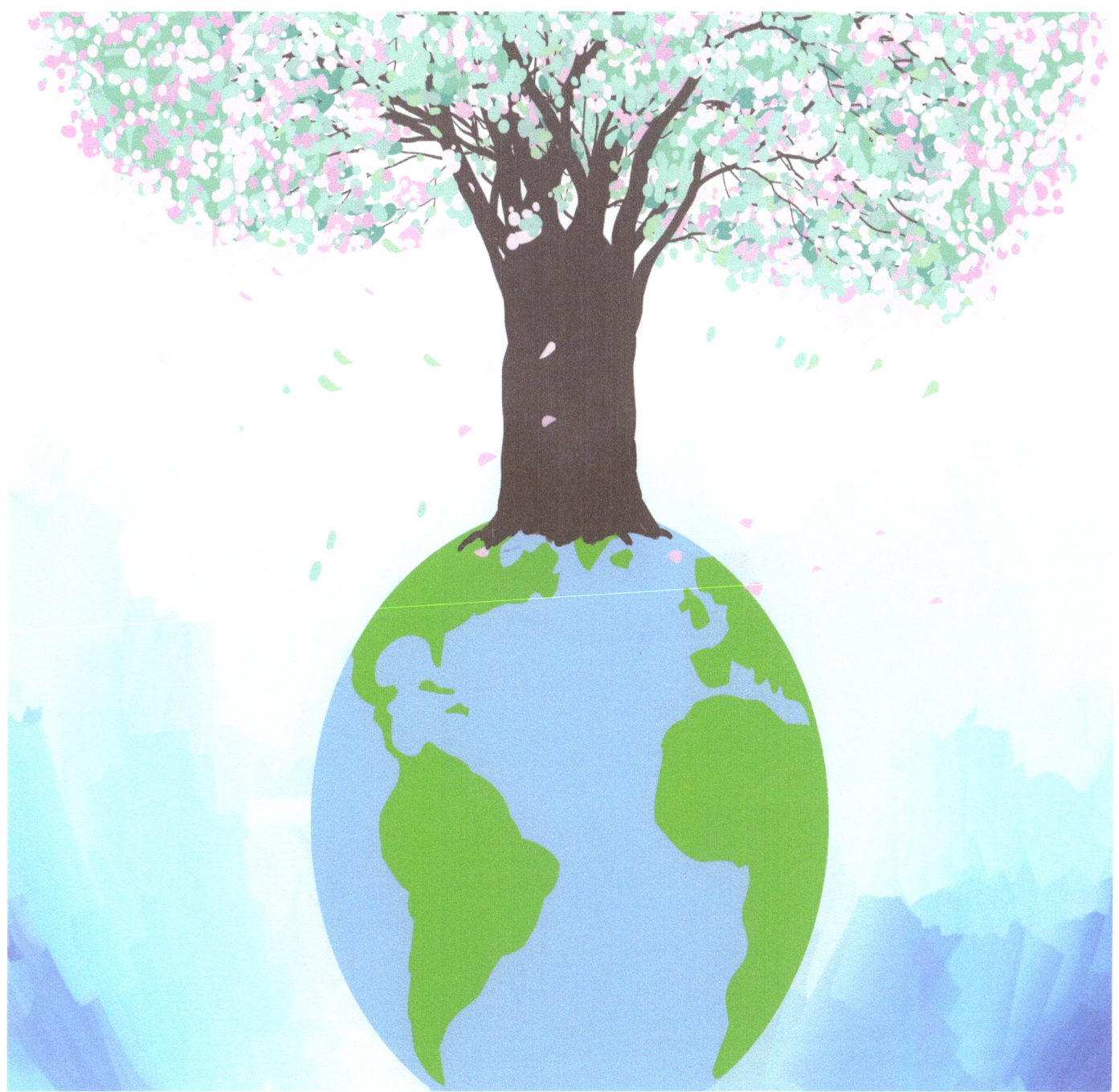

To Parents and Caregivers:

The Loving Kindness meditation has been practiced by parents and children around the world for many generations. This meditation has an instantly positive effect on oneself and others. When praticed regularly it may provide the tools to navigate through stressful situations, whether during the teenage years or adult life.